The Porn Guru

A Guide to Stop Porn Dependency

Also Includes:

30 Days to Quit Porn

Copyright © JV 2021

Share this book and help others!

Now that you're on the journey toward a porn-free life, you'll encounter more inner and outer peace. Porn takes a toll on the mind and causes dependency that eventually leads to a negative trajectory. It's time to break that unneeded chain!

Help others by posting a picture of this book's cover (or the link) on social media and including #ThePornGuru and #NoPorn along with any hashtags you believe would help spread awareness. The benefits of a porn-free life should be experienced by everyone. May you have an enlightened perspective of sex, an awakened mind, and an abundance of peace in your heart!

This book is meant to be a guide only. If the lessons and exercises in this book are followed, relief can happen. This guide is not meant to substitute professional treatment when needed.

The last half of the book consists of a 30-day mindfulness program that can be used in conjunction with the primary chapters.

If interested in a more reality-therapy and satirical approach to self-help, look for the book "You Suck" by Paulie Amigo.

Check out more helpful books at www.30DaysNow.com or search for Harper Daniels and Corin Devaso on Amazon.

Contents

Preface 5

Chapter 1: What's the Problem? 7
Chapter 2: The Great Orgasm 14
Chapter 3: Awareness and Observation 18
Chapter 4: Blind to Reality 26
Chapter 5: The Never Ending Fantasy 30
Chapter 6: Imagine Being a Porn Star 33
Chapter 7: Trapped in Your Mind 36
Chapter 8: The Fulfilled and Free Life 38

30 Days to Quit Porn 40
Day 1 42
Day 2 43
Day 3 44
Day 4 45
Day 5 46
Day 6 47
Day 7 48
Day 8 49
Day 9 50
Day 10 51
Day 11 52
Day 12 53
Day 13 54
Day 14 55
Day 15 56
Day 16 57
Day 17 58
Day 18 59
Day 19 60
Day 20 61
Day 21 62
Day 22 63
Day 23 64
Day 24 65
Day 25 66

Day 26	67
Day 27	68
Day 28	69
Day 29	70
Day 30	71
Conclusion	72

Preface

From the outset, I'll be straight with you...don't read this book if you think it's going to save you from an addiction and revolutionize your life. If your life does change for the better after reading this book, it's only because you woke up and allowed change to occur. This book is only a guide to help you understand and drop a habit. In the case of this small book, the habit is none other than pornography dependence. Please keep in mind, this book is neither anti nor pro-pornography. It's not meant to be a religious book or a rallying cry to save people from pornography addiction. If you're looking for an author, group, or mission to preach against pornography, just search the internet and you'll find plenty; but this guide is not that.

This book takes a different approach to help people understand and address a common habit. You may not even be dependent on pornography - perhaps you're simply curious about pornography dependence, or maybe you're reading this book because you wish to help a friend or loved one with a strong attachment to porn. It doesn't matter why you're reading this book; I just ask that you keep an open mind.

Some of the material you may find offensive. The topic of pornography is considered risqué, but for the purpose of this book, try to see it as normal as a dependence on coffee – coffee addiction has become normalized, similar to porn's normalization. The goal of this guide isn't to fight this normalized and universal dependency. The bottom line: this book doesn't intend to take sides, exhort, judge, or tell you what to do or not to do. Simply relax, read, question, and most importantly...self observe.

If you keep an open mind, I'm confident you'll gain a lot from this book. If your life improves even ten percent from having read this short guide, that's a huge accomplishment. Also, keep in mind that real change is often uncomfortable and sometimes painful; so if you follow the advice in this book and experience rough and unpleasant emotions, then that's a good sign you're starting to wake up and ready to drop a pernicious dependency.

(The last portion of this book is a 30-day mindfulness program that you can follow to drop an attachment to porn. The lessons and exercise in the 30-day program can also be applied to other dependencies.)

Help others by posting a picture of this book's cover (or the link) on social media and including #ThePornGuru and #NoPorn along with any hashtags you believe would help spread awareness. The benefits of a porn-free life should be experienced by everyone. May you have an enlightened perspective of sex, an awakened mind, and an abundance of peace in your heart!

Chapter 1

What's the Problem?

It's often the case that people with a pornography dependency aren't aware of the reason why they're watching actors bang for bucks. They just know that something about porn arouses them to orgasm or feeds a mental craving, but they can't pinpoint one primary factor about the video or image that excites their senses.

One guy might say it's watching young naked women ride each other that gives him an erection; yet another guy needs to watch an Asian girl dressed like a housemaid bouncing reverse on an old bloke. For women, one woman might say she needs her porn to include a black guy and white guy teaming up on a brunette; while another woman requires her porn to include a geyser climax from the female actor. If these scenarios seem absurd or offensive, you're going to have a difficult time reading this book. Those scenarios are mild compared to what's sailing on the vast ocean of internet pornography.

In these examples, it seems like these viewers know what they want; like preferring different toppings on a pizza. But have they always enjoyed such specific porn, or have their preferences changed throughout the years? These are just examples, but the answer is both: some people spend their entire lives drawn to one specific kind of pornography, but even more peoples' taste in porn evolves into something far distant to what they initially favored. Nevertheless, it's not just one thing that causes porn dependency. It can be quite complicated, because we as people are very complicated, especially our sexuality. So the question is…what's the problem? Remember, this book is neither anti-porn nor pro-porn; it's to simply help you become aware of the reasons behind porn dependency; in other words, to wake you up (or give you the tools to help a friend wake up) from reliance on porn.

To determine if porn is causing you a problem, you'll need to be honest with yourself. Let's back up just a bit. First, you'll need to define the problem or your criteria for determining if you have a problem. Later on we'll get into psychological costs, risks, and health; but for now, consider whether or not you are living happily with porn. Happiness is what everyone wants, all day and every day. Porn is either adding or subtracting from your happiness; so which is it? I'm not going to define happiness, as that's something not easily definable; however, the consensus is that peace, contentment, fulfillment, gratitude, and love accompany a happy life.

Have you ever heard people say that addicts use porn to fill a happiness void? That's probably bullshit. I don't know you, so I can't determine if porn adds or subtracts to your baseline happiness. There's no way to know if you have some deep and dark void that is being filled with porn. Do you honestly think a void in your life can be filled with a video of two people licking each other's genitals? I'm going to give you much more credit than that; I believe you're aware enough to realize that pornography can't fill a happiness void.

I just ask that you be honest with yourself, and ask if you're dependent on porn at some level of attachment. If you are, it's more than likely subtracting from your baseline happiness, because no level of dependency is healthy. Some smartass may be thinking, *"Well, that doesn't make sense. We need to be dependent on certain things. Like water, food, heat, money, and sex!"* Let's be clear, we're not talking about the absolute necessities for human life. We're talking about actors getting sloppy with each other to make a quick grand, get out of credit card or student loan debt, or find a way onto the Hollywood scene…which most porn stars never do by the way.

If you're not certain if you're dependent on porn, or if you don't know the intensity of your dependency, do this – go two months without pornography. If it gives you pause to even consider going so long without looking at images of naked humans smashing each other crazy style, then you probably have a problem with porn. Maybe you can easily go for two months without using pornography; then you may not have a problem. And if you can go for two months without pornography and not experience anxiety, depression, irritation, sleeplessness, anger, or any type of emotional rollercoaster, then close this book and start your porn-free journey right now.

However, if you know in your gut that you won't make it two weeks without craving a video of a nude person screaming *"Yes! Yes! No!",* or whatever your porn forte is, then there's a problem. But that's not to say you're weird or doomed to be porn dependent forever. Define and confront the problem now before you become too complacent.

Now back to the examples above. As mentioned, it's never one specific aspect of a porn image or video that arouses someone. There's typically a narrative involved. Why do you think there are so many porn videos on the internet? Rarely do people view images of genitalia only, or whatever excites them (*I won't apologize for the language, and it'll probably get much worse or funny, depending on your filter*). It's a smorgasbord of parts and sounds that people want and demand. One person wants a salad bar with fruit, but another prefers a seafood buffet – it's the same with porn, everyone has a specific liking, so producers are constantly working to appease various tastes. Why do you think porn is such a lucrative business for adult entertainment companies? The diversity in porn allows for never-ending streams of profit.

So, what type of porn arouses you? What types of images, stories, sounds, and body types excite you; and in what combinations? Which pictures and videos do you regularly return to; and have you moved on to different kinds? If there has been a change in the porn you view, what exactly changed and when? Take some time and think about these questions. Write down your answers on a piece of paper if needed, and then place the piece of paper in your neighbor's mailbox (*that was a joke, and I'm not to blame if you do that*).

The point is: you must become aware of the specifics of your dependency. Pornography itself is not the problem; your dependency is. For example, someone might say, "*I'm dependent on pornography, it takes up most of my leisure time*," but are they referring to all pornography, or a specific kind – such as robust German men mounting each other like blonde unicorns? Almost always, a person with a dependency is drawn to specific things. This applies to much more than pornography. Only you can determine if you have a real problem with porn, even a slight one; and only you can drop the problem at any time. A problem does not have to be a stressful dilemma. In fact, problems are great teachers.

When I was a teenager, I remember helping a family friend move. This family friend developed a terrible brain disease that eventually led to his immobility. He lost his ability to speak and move - it was a terrible situation to witness.

However, I remember on the day we were helping him move, he was sitting in a room watching porn. Barely able to move, and unable to speak well, he used pornography to excite his senses – not because he wanted to, but because he was conditioned. All the years he spent viewing pornography led to a severe dependency; so severe that porn was one of the last things he was holding on to. In the end, he wasn't able to operate a toaster, but he could order porn on his television. The nurses were amazed. This story isn't meant to scare or depress you. The point of the story is to show you that dependency is a real problem, and it can, and often does, evolve in strange ways if left alone. It was too late for the family friend to learn the lesson, but it was a great lesson for those who witnessed the problem. Porn can, and often does, lead to strange actions.

I previously mentioned a similarity between coffee and porn, but now I'll change gears and tell you that there are obvious differences. The most important difference is that porn dependency is unique, and the uniqueness involves the narrative. Why is it that my family friend continued to watch porn even though he couldn't get any physical benefit from it? I'm referring to the orgasm. Ever wonder that? Why would older men, unable to have an erection, without the ability to have an orgasm, be addicted to porn? The same question applies to some older women. The simple answer is: the brain is a very powerful computer. If the brain is wired and coded in a particular way, it's nearly impossible to change; and when the brain is wired for a particular narrative, it'll seek it in bizarre ways and will do anything to obtain it. By "narrative" I'm referring to the stories told through porn.

Does this mean there's no hope and you'll be dependent on porn forever, assuming you do have an ongoing habit? While you might depend on porn, the answer to that question depends on you. If left on a small desert island without any technology, would you still be dependent on porn after a few months? Probably not. However, you don't have the luxury to do away with your computer, Smartphone, tablet, and television. So, is the answer to fight the problem until your brain rewires? I'll save you a lot of headaches by telling you that is not the answer; in fact, fighting a dependency as strong as porn can lead to some strange outcomes.

I remember attending a debate between a famous porn star and a porn producer turned evangelist. The redeemed porn producer dedicated his new life to fighting the porn industry and preaching against porn use; it made sense at the time. Years later, the redeemed producer was arrested on felony sex charges. If you spend a lot of time and energy fighting something, you often become intimately involved with it. Whatever you do, don't fight dependency. You won't win that fight.

So, realize that porn is not the problem. The problem is the dependency, and the dependency is in the dependent. That's why it's important to think about the questions posed earlier. In other words, get to know your dependency. I'm confident that if you see it for what it truly is, you'll then lose the desire to use pornography. It won't matter to you any longer.

Points to Ponder:
(You can share chapter insights, advice, and thoughts online using #PornGuruProblem)

How long can you go without using, viewing, or thinking about pornography?

Are you reliant on pornography to some degree?

It's important to define what it is that you're dependent on. What are the specific sights and sounds of porn that you regularly desire? Why do you think you're dependent on those specific narratives?

Any degree of dependency is too much. We are not built to be dependent on porn. It's not sustainable or healthy, and this external sexual dependency can evolve into irregular conditioning.

Porn is not the problem. Dependency is the problem.

The problem is in you; as you maintain the dependency.

Don't fight a desire or dependency with willpower. You'll lose the fight.

Chapter 2

The Great Orgasm

One of the most powerful, intense, and energetic reactions in nature is the human orgasm. The human race depends on this extreme reaction. Sounds silly, right? But it's true. If you've ever had an orgasm, you know what I mean. It feels like a mix between profound pain and profound pleasure – pleasure and pain are two sides of the same coin by the way. So, why is there a chapter on orgasms? And what does this have to do with porn dependency?

Any dependency you have - whether it's using pornography, smoking cigarettes, or checking your Smartphone ever three minutes – feeds on a reward and pleasure system. It doesn't matter how mild the dependency. All dependencies are based on attachments to pleasures, and those attachments exist because of feelings that cause dynamic chemical reactions in your brain. I'm not going to get into the science, but I do recommend you research brain chemicals when you have a moment. Neurochemistry is a very interesting topic, and studying it, even a little bit, can bring a much-needed understanding of your habits.

Every time you have an orgasm an extremely powerful chemical called dopamine is released in your brain. This is like a shot of heroin, no joke. It's natural and totally fine; whereas heroin can kill you after making your life into a living hell. Not to single out heroin as a killer drug – methamphetamine and fentanyl are also killers, and they too spike dopamine to intense levels. Essentially, having an orgasm is like taking a powerful synthetic drug that fills your brain and body with wonderful sensations that are driven by dopamine. Again, to be clear: orgasms are safe and healthy, synthetic drugs are not. The point is to awaken you to the power and intensity of the orgasm. The orgasm has a truly remarkable effect on your brain and body; mostly due to natural brain chemicals such as dopamine, as mentioned.

Though the orgasm is a healthy force that we depend on to continue populating the planet – you wouldn't be alive and reading this without an orgasm having happened – it can also be the cause of peculiar dependencies, namely sexual, that can be detrimental to our well-being. In other words, if something as powerful as an orgasm can be associated with a sight, sound, touch, taste, or combination of these, then an unhealthy and unnatural association can develop. In the case of porn, we're talking about sight, sound, possibly touch, and hopefully not taste, unless you lick your mobile device or computer while viewing porn, which would be unusually weird. Naturally, it's sight, sound, touch, and taste during actual sex, in comparison to virtual sex, that arouses the mind and body to orgasm. Porn use interrupts that instinct and redirects the association.

This is basic information. Think about any dependency you have, and ask yourself, *"What is the pleasure associated with this?"* What pleasure does the alcoholic get from the intoxication? What pleasure does the smoker get from the cigarette? What pleasure does the worker get from his job, even though he may despise doing it? What pleasure do you get from eating food? Smoking cigarettes and eating food are different dependencies – one is healthy, and one isn't - but eating food is a natural dependency for basic survival, whereas no living creature needs a cigarette for sustenance and survival. Have you ever seen a squirrel smoking a cigarette? The point is: whatever the dependency, regardless of unhealthy or healthy, there's going to be a pleasure associated with it. For the purpose of this book, consider emotional and relational dependencies as unhealthy; and physical dependencies, such as food and shelter, as healthy. In essence, discover and understand the pleasure behind the dependency, as well as the tool you use to deliver that pleasure.

Porn is a tool for arousing one's self sexually. Regardless of whether or not you believe in evolution, can you think of any other mammal that uses a tool to cause an orgasm? The animal kingdom is free, open, and wild...without porn. Watch nature, it just does its own thing, without the aid of a sexual tool. When an animal must have sex, it either does or does not. If it looks for a mate but can't find one, it doesn't die – the animal simply moves on. But people who are dependent on porn to have an orgasm do not move on. Typically, the dependency strengthens, until the person seeks out new pornographic material. Even if a person does wear himself or herself out on pornography, the person usually returns to it sooner or later; because as mentioned, they've associated the powerful effect of the orgasm with a specific sight and sound of the video or picture. I'll say it again; orgasms are healthy and are not the problem. The problem is developing an association. The problem is the dependency.

So, if a person has already developed an association between the intense sensation of the orgasm and porn, how does the person break the dependency? The answer is: by not breaking it; but instead, by dropping the attachment. And the only way to drop a dependency of any intensity is through awareness and self-observation.

Points to Ponder:
(You can share chapter insights, advice, and thoughts online using #PornGuruOrgasm)

The orgasm is a release of intense energy. It is neither good nor bad, but it is simply a powerful reaction that causes euphoric feelings throughout the body and mind.

Associating the energy and euphoric effects of orgasm with something such as porn can lead to a strong dependency. This will cause unawareness and unhappiness. In other words; this dependency takes away from your natural ability to orgasm and feel free.

Don't be ashamed of orgasms. They are necessary for life. Drop the association between porn and orgasm. If you have orgasms while using pornography, you are reinforcing an unnatural association.

Let orgasms happen naturally, without the use of porn; and if you cannot have an orgasm without the use of porn, then be content with no orgasm.

Don't associate or define your "self" with the orgasm, or absence of it.

Like most things, the orgasm comes and goes. You're happiness and presence is not dependent on its occurrence. Whether or not you experience one, does not matter. You can be happy regardless.

Chapter 3

Awareness and Observation

Let's say you've determined that you're dependent on porn, and you already identified the specifics of your dependency; then, how do you go about addressing the dependency if you can't fight or escape it? The answer is simple, but most people find it incredibly difficult to apply. I'm talking about awareness and observation. This is the only way to overcome a strong dependency for good.

Fighting an addiction, no matter how mild it may be, often fuels it in the long term. I'm sure you know someone who is a recovering addict of alcohol, cigarettes, or other drugs. How long has that person remained free from the addiction…a year, five years, or maybe ten years? It's often the case that relapse occurs; and when it does, the dependency is stronger than ever. It's not that the relapsed addict is weak, heartless, or incapable of being free from the vice once and for all. The issue is that recovering addicts still identify as addicts, and with that identity comes the belief that they'll need to fight the dependency for their entire lives. Does that sound like happiness to you? Does that sound like freedom? Real freedom is dropping something without fighting and walking away without regret or remorse. When you make something your enemy, you're joined to it forever.

This is the reason why this book isn't anti-porn. To be anti-anything doesn't help to drop a dependency. Giving any thought (even an adversarial thought) to something pleasurable, such as pornography, only serves the habit, not you. So, don't fight your addiction, dependency, habit, or whatever you wish to call it; but neither accept it as part of you, because it's not. Simply be aware of its influence in your life, be mindful of the specifics as mentioned in the previous chapter, and observe your thoughts without judgment.

This is difficult to do when starting out, but with a little time and practice, you can make great strides in dropping your porn habit. In fact, if you viewed porn today, or plan on using porn later, don't let me stop you. This isn't a message to fight or restrain. As mentioned, don't associate the dropping of a dependency with conflict. Remember, fighting a craving will only give it power in the long term. Willpower works for the short-term, until you fail or become an irritable asshole. So, the best way to let go of a dependency is through awareness and observation of the dependency and the specifics involved.

Let's do an exercise:

Can you tell me what your next thought will be? What will you be thinking five minutes from now? Can you know for certain what your next three or four thoughts will be? Seriously ponder these questions.

You can make an educated guess, but odds are you'll have no clue what thoughts will enter your head today, let alone in the next two minutes. And if you can't know for certain what your next thoughts will be, or what emotions will arise from those thoughts, do you have any control over them?

You may have a controlled response to certain thoughts, such as remaining calm when you experience anger at a friend's lack of respect, but could you prevent the angry thought from manifesting? Take ten minutes and ask yourself, *"What will be the next couple of thoughts and emotions I'll experience?"*

You may have felt a blankness or uncertainty during that exercise; and if so, wonderful. That is self-observation. You were thoughtless and observing, without judgment. There really isn't much more to it; however, this is not an easy thing to practice, because we tend to have an insatiable need to be in control and would rather remain hypnotized by random thoughts. In other words, we would rather believe we're in control of thoughts; and that's like saying the sky is in control of clouds, which it is not. Thoughts, even sexual thoughts, are simply clouds passing through the mind. What you just practiced is a form of mindfulness. Observe the thoughts coming and going through your mind. (The last part of this book includes a 30-day mindfulness program that you can practice.)

By asking, *"What will my next thought be?"* you're essentially getting out of your own head for a few minutes. This can often feel like a mini-vacation, especially if you experience wildly fluctuating thoughts all day long; or it can cause you anxiety if you're the type of person who demands control. This leads to another question: *are you separate from your thoughts*?

You might be thinking, *"Is this author a Buddhist?"* Not necessarily; but I do believe that mindfulness is a great way to become aware and drop a dependency. Observation and mindfulness combined can work wonders for all types of dependencies, especially strong ones such as pornography. If you're living an unobserved life, you're missing out on a lot. Though the brain is a powerful computer hard wired to think in particular patterns, it does not want to be dependent on something like pornography, because there is no long term health benefit.

As strong as they feel at times, sexual desires are not part of your identity. They are simply desires, which are born of thoughts. Most people are raised and conditioned by family and society to believe that certain sexual lusts are necessary for a particular identity. It's not uncommon to hear about certain fathers who purposefully leave pornography around the house in hopes that their sons will find it and develop a desire for naked women. Many of those fathers do this to influence their sons' sexuality. That practice may not be as prevalent today since porno magazines are a thing of the past, but you get the point. It's also common for young girls to find their fathers' or siblings' porn, and thus develop an idea of what's expected of them as women – i.e. what a woman should look like, behave as, and be comfortable with. The point: you, as a unique individual, are not thoughts or desires. At your core, you are free, like the blue sky.

However, the goal of the porn industry, the porn producers, the porn actors, and all the businesses involved in the production of pornography, is to make you believe that your identity is intimately associated with an image or video. Consider the marketing: *"Click now to see this. You want to see this," "I'll fulfill your fantasy," "I'll do anything you want me to do," "Don't you want to see me do this."* It's all directed at "you" – the "you" that they know you've been conditioned to be and believe. From a business perspective, it's brilliant and sustainable, because adult entertainment companies know that most people are unaware and nonobservant. Porn offers people an identity, though illusory.

As another example, consider a heterosexual guy who walks up to his peer and shows him a video of an attractive red-head female being gang-banged by a group of men. Most of the time, the friend will feel a strong obligation to respond favorably, such as, *"Wow! That's awesome," "I wish I was there," "She's hot"*, or a similar response, even though the friend may be disturbed by the video. The friend knows that if he has no reaction or reacts with disgust, then his sexuality will be in question. Not all heterosexual guys feel obligated to respond in those ways, but the vast majority do, simply because of the pressure to maintain a conditioned sexual identity. This idea also applies to other sexual orientations as well. It's rare that someone can drop their dependency on conditioned sexual identity; it takes a lot of courage to do that without reacting.

Consider one more example of people using sexual thoughts and desires to reinforce an illusory identity. Many people feel that they have to masturbate often to be deemed a healthy individual, and some go so far as to think a trophy is warranted for masturbating consecutive times per day. This is not to say masturbation is wrong – that's not the point here – but the idea that one's identity is dependent on the frequency or ability to masturbate keeps the person from present moment awareness. Some women and men will express embarrassment for not being able to masturbate, and on the other hand (which is hopefully clean) some women and men will think they're sexual rock stars for masturbating two or three times daily. Again, the point is not to judge masturbation one way or the other, but to help you realize that masturbation has nothing to do with your identity or worth. However, porn will have you think otherwise; because the porn industry is heavily dependent on people masturbating to image, audio, and visual.

Let's get back to observation. By now, you should be aware that you're not to blame for compulsory thoughts or desires that cause dependency. With that said, you are responsible for how you respond to them; and as mentioned, struggling against them, or trying hard to lessen their frequency, won't help. Going back to the lesson about thought observance, ask yourself, *"What stories do my sexual thoughts tell?"* What part do you play in the stories? What part does the other person, or persons, play? Don't intensely analyze these thoughts, and don't judge them as good or bad, just observe. When you consider the answers to these questions, do you feel any emotions? Which emotions? Again, you must be in a state of mind to look at these things objectively, without judgment. Observe the thoughts and emotions you experience.

Now, how does porn reinforce these stories? What images, videos, or audio do you use to make these whimsical stories more real in your mind? Do you see how the illusion takes hold and begins to affect your mind?

Here's an exercise:

Observe your thoughts and feelings before, during, and after porn use. Write down your observations if you are able to. Don't try to stop or prevent thoughts or feelings, just let them happen as normal, and take note of what's going on inside you; that is, what you're experiencing in thought and emotion. What thoughts come into your mind before, during, and immediately after viewing or masturbating to porn?

During this entire process, observe your breathing, muscle movements, movement of your eyes, and the sounds you might make. Also, pay attention to what you do after using porn – do you sleep, exercise, study, watch television, go to work, etc? Again, it'll help if you write down your observations. Think of it like you're observing a totally different person without judgment.

Observation is a quick way to awareness. Few people are capable of observing their thoughts and emotions objectively, but you can do this. Think of this like going to the gym, but for your mind. When you observe the thoughts and feelings you have before, during, and after porn use, the dependency will weaken. It's important to remember not to strain or fight; instead, simply observe, like you would clouds passing through the sky or cars passing on a highway.

Wake up and realize that you are not dependent on porn, and you never were. You were easily conditioned, at no fault of your own, to believe porn is helpful for establishing and maintaining a sexual identity. It is not. Porn keeps you unaware. Through observation, you can wake up and live free of its dependency. In essence, you are not actually dependent on porn; it, however, is dependent on you.

Points to Ponder:
(You can share chapter insights, advice, and thoughts online using #PornGuruAwareness)

Awareness and observation are the way to drop a dependency.

Never fight a dependency; fighting makes you intimately involved with it.

The being you call "you" is not constructed by sexual thoughts, desires, or lusts. "You" are completely independent of those, despite what your family, society, and culture teach.

Sexual thoughts are neither good nor bad; they're simply clouds passing through the blue sky of your mind. Let them pass.

Porn would have you believe that your sexual thoughts and desires are stronger than they really are and that you must obey them. That is a lie. For porn to be a profitable business, it needs you to believe this deception.

Observe your thoughts, reactions, feelings, and emotions before, during, and after using pornography. If possible, write them down. Do this without judgment; simply observe.

You are not dependent on having or maintaining a sexual identity, especially one reinforced by porn. Be one of the awakened few who are completely free from constructed identity.

Chapter 4

Blind to Reality

If you don't have a quiet mind, life can be difficult. Think of all the distractions in our modern world that prevent a quiet mind: social media, cable, email, apps, blogs, smartphones…the list is endless. Never before have there been so many toys to distract us from reality. If you lose your smartphone, you might have a panic attack. Something is wrong, but it doesn't have to be.

People are unable to accept reality; as a result, anxiety and depression are on the rise because we've forgotten that we exist in biological bodies - we're not robots, even though our technological tools condition us to believe we are. Since you're in a flesh and blood body, there are certain conditions you need to obtain maximal wellbeing. One of those conditions is to be grounded in offline reality, not virtual or online reality. So the question is: what is reality?

By reading this far, you know that reality is not found in porn; or to stay it differently…porn is not reality. So where do you find reality? And why should you listen to me, or anyone else for that matter, in your quest to find *the real*? Without going too deep into philosophy, let's just say that you cannot experience reality if you are dependent on something such as porn. Whatever is real, porn blinds you to it; and it blinds you by fogging a quiet and still mind.

Porn addicts believe that pornography assists with quieting their minds and relieving stress; but what they're actually experiencing is the aftermath of an orgasm; which as mentioned earlier feels relaxing and calming, as it's an intense energy that releases powerful neurochemicals. However, if the addict doesn't have an orgasm, the person will still feel relief because the false identity was affirmed and the sexual illusion was fed; similar to a screaming cat becoming quiet after it's been given a can of tuna. To be clear, though it appears to the porn dependent person that the mind is calm and relaxed, it isn't. It's simply in a deeper state of disillusionment.

The magic of porn consists in its ability to blind you to the reality of the present, and you are part of the present moment. The producers of porn work hard to create fantasies that draw you out of reality and into a false narrative. Not only that, but they also want to keep you there, even when you're not viewing porn. The goal for every adult entertainment business is to have you keep coming back for more…more delusion, sexual affirmation, and fabricated identity. Essentially, the goal of porn is to tell you that there's a better reality, and a better you, and it's found in porn. Wake up, and see that it's a lie. Life is too short to be lived in fantasy.

Here's an exercise:

Reality is here and now. If you're reading this, look up and tell me what you see. Turn off your phone, or whatever distraction you're using, and sit or stand quietly for ten minutes observing and listening. Even if you're in an empty room without much color or action, simply look and listen. If you're finding this difficult, concentrate on your breathing, listen to it. Touch the desk in front of you. Clap your hands together once. Listen, observe, and feel. This is reality. Silence and stillness are the gateways to the real.

An experience like that can be frightening to many people because what occurs is this: you become aware of yourself, and the self is what we tend to fear most. Porn offers an escape from having to learn about yourself, especially how you react to sexual experiences. It can be incredibly frightening for someone who's been dependent on porn to drop the dependency and experience reality; but just like the clouds mentioned earlier, that fright will pass by and out of sight.

When a person steps away from a porn dependency into the present moment, new and wonderful things are discovered. A lovely feeling of security, an increase in confidence, and inner peace are experienced. The person may feel a pullback toward using porn, but that will pass with time. The next step after this new awaking is to experience sex in reality.

Sex does not have to be complex or goal-oriented. Porn makes it seem like sex always has some grandiose goal and involves a complex process, but that's not reality. For example, take the run-of-the-mill porn film: two strangers meet unexpectedly and through a series of carefully constructed lame conversations they end up doing naked gymnastics – flipping, bending, pounding, smashing, and flexing with Olympic style accuracy; and in the end, there's an earth-shattering orgasm. How often do you think that occurs in reality?

Instead of experiencing sex in reality and seeing the authenticity of real physical intimacy, people who regularly use porn see an illusion that blinds them to the truth. It's much easier to remain asleep and dreaming, than wake up; which is why dropping porn can bring on agitation and frustration at first. The point is: it is better for you to wake up from your porn illusion and experience sex when it occurs in reality, without any grandiose expectations or goals. By the way, do you actually think there's someone on the planet who can give you prodigious orgasms on a regular basis?

Points to Ponder:
(You can share chapter insights, advice, and thoughts online using #PornGuruReality)

Porn distracts the mind from seeing and experiencing reality.

Though it seems like porn clears the mind of stress and agitation, it does the opposite. It's a temporary relief, and it drives the person into a deeper state of disillusionment.

The goal of porn is to blind you to the present moment and keep you from experiencing and enjoying real sex, which is not at all like porn.

Waking up from a disillusion can be painful, frustrating, and agitating; but it's better than remaining asleep in a fog. The pain, frustration, and agitation will pass like a cloud, and a balance will be restored to your mind and soul.

Chapter 5

The Never Ending Fantasy

Ask yourself, *"How many clicks will it take for me to be satisfied?"* Have you ever thought of that? Let's look at this objectively: how many porn views, mouse clicks, smartphone taps, and downloads will it take for a person dependent on porn to reach ultimate gratification? After all, what's the end goal?

The nature of pornography is to keep you believing that there's an achievable end goal. These mass-produced sexual fantasies are sending the messages, *"Keep looking and using, because this is what you can have someday," "You want this, and we'll give it to you. All you need to do is continue watching,"* and *"You can easily be in this fantasy. You're capable of playing the role. You are sexy for even watching this. This can be yours in reality."* By watching porn, you are hypnotizing yourself; and hypnosis can feel real. It's all a trick of the mind, reinforced by the great and powerful orgasm, as previously talked about.

Not only is it hypnosis, but it's also a psychological cyclone that evolves into obscure dependencies. The most popular porn fantasies on the internet – meaning, the porn that receives the most views and downloads – involve the words "teen", "stepmom", "hentai", "gangbang", "creampie", and other narrative-based terms. Have you ever wondered how someone can go from watching two grown adults smashing to watching an older adult screw a teenager in a video titled *Student, Girl Next Door,* or *Stepdaughter*? Or going from watching two lesbians make out, to an animated hentai gangbang?

The reason for this evolution in porn dependency is none other than the narrative of the film or image. The user of porn is dependent on a story, not just seeing two naked people shag. There's a deeper meaning; and stronger hypnosis. And unlike real stories, the stories of pornography don't have endings...besides explosive orgasms. What results is a dependency that feeds on itself, always looking for the end; but the final act never comes. Porn does not let the viewer leave with a feeling of true contentment and fulfillment; if it did, the porn industry wouldn't be worth billions of dollars. And if you think porn does result in a feeling of fulfillment, you're mistaking orgasmic neurochemicals for emotional satisfaction.

Why porn terms such as *teen* and *stepmom* are so prevalent speaks more to a narrative than it does to the desire to see naked people get nasty. So, what narrative do you desire? What do the people in your porn fantasy look like, what are their roles, what are they doing, how are they behaving, where are they smashing, and what role in the narrative are you identifying with? Observe the narratives that you are drawn to and have developed a dependency on. Also, ask yourself how these narratives have evolved over time and how they relate to your real life. Use these questions to reflect and learn about your conditioning.

Porn and Disney have more in common than you might think: fantasy and manipulation by means of narrative. However, as destructive as Snow White may be to the emotional and cognitive development of little girls and boys; that story doesn't cause the catastrophic destruction of porn that depicts her being gangbanged by the Seven Dwarfs. Porn is a fantasy that is reinforced by the powerful neurochemicals of your amazingly powerful human brain. It's a fantasy you don't want to entertain.

Points to Ponder:
(You can share chapter insights, advice, and thoughts online using #PornGuruFantasy)

The fantasy of porn does not have an ending. Though it may feel like orgasm is the ultimate ending and purpose, it is not; on the contrary, the climax creates a growing and insatiable desire for more of the story.

You will never be able to see, click, scroll through, or download enough porn. There is never enough. There is no ending. Either you will forever utilize porn and become increasingly insensitive and sexually manipulated, or you will drop the dependency completely and live without the attachment.

Porn is a form of hypnosis. It's time to wake up. How long do you wish to remain asleep? Wake up already!

If you think, "*Watching a few hot naked people bang isn't that bad. Everybody watches porn, and not everybody is a sexual maniac,*" then you're making an excuse and overlooking the fact that porn has evolved, and continues to evolve, into uniquely specific narratives that more and more people are craving. Remember those popular trending titles: *Dad Does Stepdaughter, Stepmom Does Son, Teenage Neighbor, Naughty Babysitter, Bad Student, etc.* If porn was a fairly safe fantasy with a clear purpose, a safe end goal, and a simple narrative, then it would not be evolving into these twisted fantasies that consumers of porn are demanding. Porn isn't a garden rose, it's a noxious weed that overtakes your imagination and puts your natural desires and inclinations to sleep.

The Seven Dwarfs had other plans.

Chapter 6

Imagine Being a Porn Star

Honestly, do you think you can act in a porn film or have photos taken of you naked? Maybe you have a lot of pride and confidence and think, *"Hell yes! I'd do porn in a heartbeat. Especially if it pays well."* Let's hope you're not that ignorant and arrogant to believe you would enjoy being filmed and told what to do. You can look porn statistics up online after reading this chapter, but I'll save you the trouble and let you know that the average career of a porn star lasts a few months, at best. And they walk away with little cash to show for having their ass cheeks spread for the world to see. Being a porn star sucks in more ways than one.

Healthy sex is supposed to be tense, awkward, intimidating, sensual, transparent, a mix of excitement and anxiety, and consensual. Now imagine adding cameras, lights, a room full of people, a director telling you what to do and what not to do, an acting partner who you've never met before and who will most likely be intoxicated, and funky smells. Never has a porn star thought, *"I really like my job. It's the greatest."* But to the porn industry, it doesn't matter if these short-lived porn stars hate their jobs and lives because the industry knows that you'll take what the producers create and form a unique fantasy. All the industry needs are young, hot, and stupid individuals who believe doing porn will help them make a million dollars, get out of student loan debt, or be a gateway into a modeling career or Hollywood.

And not all porn stars are stupid, as there are many stories of people getting into porn by means of manipulation: i.e.

made to do porn in order to pay off a debt, lied to and told their photos won't be put online, needing quick cash to feed a drug addiction, or to please a pimp. Many young people are also tricked into signing "modeling" contracts, only later to find out that their contracts included having to do porn. When they try to get out of the contract, they're threatened with severe penalties and then sweet-talked into doing a few scenes.

Imagine showing up to do a few modeling shots, which you may or may not have known were nudes, to find two guys with huge dicks and a room full of various production personnel. Your modeling agent sits you down and explains that your contract included terms that relate to pornography and you are expected to perform at least two scenes. You start crying. There's a long table behind you with every type of alcohol you can imagine, a few joints, and a bowl of pills. You're told to think carefully about your next move because there are "serious repercussions" for backing out of a legal contract. You're stuck, threatened, and alone. You might think, "*I'll just get drunk and high off this stuff on the table, go numb, and hope for the best.*" After all, your agent is there and he has your best interests in mind…right?

Don't let the fantasy fool you. What you're watching are real people who aren't having sex. What you're watching is not real sex, it's important that you are awakened to this truth. Do you really think these actors and actresses (*it's difficult to call them this because they don't typically have acting experience or training*) believe they're having sex? The guys are simply trying to maintain erections and the girls are trying to follow what the directors are ordering them to do. This is why many ex-porn stars have a difficult time having real, enjoyable, authentic sex again.

Points to Ponder:
(You can share chapter insights, advice, and thoughts online using #PornGuruImagine)

However much you believe that you can do what a porn star does…you can't. This isn't a challenge, dare, or insult. You should be grateful that you can't do what they do. As long as you drop your porn dependency and stop using porn entirely, then you have a chance at experiencing real, authentic sex again.

Looks are deceiving. What appears to be two, or multiple, people having a great sexual experience are actually people who don't know each other, don't want to be there, and are there for one reason…cash.

If you have watched a lot of porn in your life thus far, you have most likely watched people, unknowingly, do porn by force, coercion, and manipulation. Guaranteed.

While watching porn, you have never watched anyone having sex. It's not sex you're watching. You're watching a performance fantasy that you're interpreting as sex. You actually have no clue what's going on. One of the greatest disasters of porn occurs when children watch porn and believe what they're viewing is real, authentic, purposeful sex.

Porn stars are not happy or proud of their work. Have you ever seen "Porn Star" or "Adult Entertainer" on a resume or career profile?

Chapter 7

Trapped In Your Mind

In the last chapter, it was stressed that viewing porn is not viewing real sex; however, you believe it is. If you never thought that porn is sexual, would you ever have viewed it, and thus become dependent on it? In other words, you have always viewed porn because you believe the illusion that you're viewing sex in some form. Sex is genuine and authentic; porn is something completely different from sex.

Can you remember the first time you saw a porn video? Whatever you thought or felt the first time is not the same as what you thought and felt the hundredth time. Why is that? The illusion evolved and created a thick wall of delusion.

Like any fantasy that is exercised over and over again, a subliminal barrier is constructed and traps you inside a pattern that believes the illusion is the real deal. Every time the illusion is employed by a porn-driven thought pattern, it is perceived as more real and authentic, though it is far removed from actual sex. You continue to view porn because your mind has been trained to discern it as real sex. Let's use a food analogy to describe this craziness:

Imagine someone tells you that a donut is an apple. At first you know it's not true, but over time you become more convinced that donuts and apples are the same. Perhaps this misperception occurs because of societal pressure, adult influence, desperation, shortage of apples, sugar addiction, manipulation, etc. Whatever the reason, you forget what an apple tastes like and you thus lose the health benefits of eating actual apples. You spend the remainder of your life indulging in donuts, believing they are nutritious apples. Of course, diabetes sets in and you suffer the consequences of a high sugar diet.

Think of porn and real sex in this way. If you continue indulging in the fantasy of porn, your mind may never be able to awaken to the experience of genuine sex ever again. And if someone attempts to have authentic sex with you, you won't recognize it and you may not even enjoy it. Sugar is highly addicting and mind-altering, as is porn. Eat real apples and have genuine sex; throw away the donuts and the porn. Free your mind from the fantasy trap.

Points to Ponder:
(You can share chapter insights, advice, and thoughts online using #PornGuruTrap)

Over time, viewing porn waters the seed of illusion. People who are dependent on porn become trapped by a subliminal barrier that won't let them experience genuine sex.

Ask yourself, *"Is porn worth losing the ability to experience authentic sex?"* Don't believe you can have both because you can't. It's either the donuts or the apples.

Your mind is incredibly powerful - more powerful than the largest computer ever created. It is a phenomenon. It has the ability to create illusion if manipulated and perceives the illusion as the real thing. However, it also has the awesome capability of repairing itself. Wake up! Porn is not real sex. You can drop the illusion at any time. Your mind is powerful enough to create the illusion and powerful enough to remove it.

Chapter 8

The Fulfilled and Free Life

This short book offered insight into a dependency that is commonplace and prevalent, but also destructive. Imagine living without the need, desire, or compulsion to view and use pornography. Even if you view porn once or twice a month, it will still be a threat to your ability to experience genuine sex, will inhibit accurate perception of self and the world, and will not add any value to your life. After all, if something doesn't add value to your life and support your life's purpose, then what is the point of entertaining the dependency?

The point of this small guide is not to abstain from pornography. Instead, the point is to awaken you to the realization that porn does not support a fulfilling and free life. Once you drop porn dependency completely (*and that goes for any dependency or adverse attachment*) then you'll forget about the need for it and will begin seeing clearly. It'll be similar to breathing fresh, clean air after having lived in a sewer for years. Once you see that you don't need, nor actually want, the fantasy of porn, you'll live a boundless life and will be more aware than you have been in a long time.

There is no benefit to porn. If you still believe there is, then review the previous chapters repeatedly (and don't forget to participate in the mindfulness program in the next part of this book) and ask yourself what the end will look like. Porn dependency, like most strong dependencies, has no plan to release you from its grip. There is no escape, end, or relief. If you continue viewing and using pornography, you may never be able to awaken to absolute awareness and enjoy the true thrills and wonders of life.

As mentioned previously, the genius of pornography is that it manipulates the amazing human mind and the powerful neurochemicals it produces. However, you do have the ability and the chance to drop the dependency instantly and allow healing to occur. The human mind and body is a master repairer; it won't be long before you see the great benefits of living a life porn-free. Drop the fantasy so you can awaken to life in the present moment. A fulfilling and free life can only occur in present moment awareness, here and now.

Points to Ponder:
(You can share chapter insights, advice, and thoughts online using #PornGuruFree)

There are no benefits to your mind and body if you continue to view and use porn. There are incredible benefits to your mind and body when you drop porn dependency.

If you want to discover or rediscover your life's purpose, then drop porn dependency as well as any adverse dependencies you are relying on for false fulfillment. Without a strong attachment to fantasy, clarity will manifest. You'll discover freedom in the present moment.

You do have the capability and intelligence to drop porn and never look back. As soon as you see it for the lie and fantasy that it is, you'll lose all desire to view and use porn.

Be excited to live the rest of your life knowing that you are free from an illusory attachment.

30 Days to Quit Porn

A 30 Day Mindfulness Program for Dropping a Porn Dependency

This next part of the guide involves a 30 day program made up of lessons and exercises to help you drop a porn dependency. Though these lessons and exercises can be applied to any unhealthy reliance, this program will focus specifically on the use of pornography.

For some readers, their dependency will drop quickly; and for others it'll drop gradually. In either case, if you stick with the program you'll start to witness your dependency weaken and you'll eventually drop it. Don't critique your progress throughout the program, as this isn't a competition and there isn't a goal you must attain. Let the dependency drop as you work through the exercises and lessons.

It's not necessary that you complete these days in order, nor should you be religious about completing them successfully. There is no such thing as a successful completion of this program. The bottom line is to observe and awaken, and that cannot be obtained through success, force, pressure, struggle, or competition. Simply relax, follow the program, and the dependency will drop.

You'll also notice that mindfulness, silence, and stillness are a regular discipline for each day. Because you've been influenced by a dependency based culture that demands instant gratification, silence and stillness may seem nearly impossible for you to practice. For this reason, we'll incorporate this discipline from the outset. A quiet and still mind is an incredibly powerful resource, but one that requires daily maintenance.

It should also be noted that you're not required to get rid of pornography that may be on your smartphone or computer; nor are you required to stop using porn if you're currently dependent on it. However, if you have already gone a few days without using porn, then it's advised that you continue without it. The point being: by practicing the following disciplines in the days to come, you won't even need willpower to drop the dependency; you can have porn right in front of you, and it won't have the slightest impact. Simply put, you'll drop all desire for porn without effort.

One of the most important lessons to keep in mind is to not fight the dependency or strive against it while participating in these exercises. If you find yourself using porn during the coming days, then that's completely fine as long as you stick to the program. Be careful not to develop a spirit of fighting or competition during this program – dependencies thrive on conflict.

You'll need about 15-30 minutes per day for the program; but feel free to spend more time if needed. The amount of time doesn't matter, as long as you're in an environment that allows you to concentrate without distraction.

One last thing: If you're like most people, you're dependent on caffeine, alcohol, or sugar to some extent. Do your best to lessen the consumption of these substances over the next 30 days. Can you cut consumption of these substances in half, or more? It's important that your mind is sober and your body relaxed to make the most of these exercises.

Let's get started.

Day 1

Exercise:

Find a place without distraction, and turn off all electronics. Sit with your back straight, kneel, or lie on a hard surface (not bed) and remain in silence for 10 minutes.

During these 10 minutes, take deep and focused breaths and hold them for a few seconds each. Exhale slowly. Listen intently to your breathing. Don't try to change it – simply listen, and feel the air go in and out.

*When you're ready, repeat the mantra: "**Be still. Be silent.**" Repeat this slowly multiple times out loud as well as quietly. You might experience boredom or anxiety, but continue repeating the mantra regardless. Repeat it until you're calm and ready. You can continue the deep breathing during the mantra, or take deep breaths during pauses. Don't rush.*

Each of the 30 days will have this time of silence, focused breathing, and a mantra. Except this page, the end of each day's page will remind you of the minutes you are to spend in silence and focused breathing for the day; and will also have a mantra for you to practice. You can repeat the mantras during your times of silence and focused breathing, or following. Remember, there is no right or wrong way to do this.

If you view porn today, practice the focused breathing and mantra before, during, and after viewing. Dependencies want to fight; in fact, they're energized by fighting. Instead of fighting the porn dependency, meet it with silence and observation. Let the exercises and lessons guide you.

Day 2

Exercise:

Ponder this question: Can you remember a time in your life when you didn't look at porn?

Writing is extremely beneficial to the mind; especially when pondering questions. Write down your thoughts about this particular question. If your mind drifts, then write whatever thoughts emerge. It's okay if you have nothing to write, but ponder the question regardless.

Were you able to remember a period in your life when you weren't using pornography? If you're like many people in western civilization, you may have to return to memories of childhood to determine that period. It's not uncommon for a person to start using porn at an early age. Some people have viewed porn before the teenage years.

Recognize that porn dependency is a learned behavior with roots. However, it's a dependency that can be dropped quickly and completely; and you have the capability to drop it.

*10 minutes of silence and focused breathing. Repeat the mantra: "**Listen and observe.**"

Day 3

Exercise:

What will your next thought be?

Try to guess what your next thought, or next two thoughts, will be.

Five minutes from now; will you be thinking about sex, work, family, a burrito, baseball, money, etc? We're not in control of our thoughts, and that scares people. We may be able to influence our thought patterns, but thoughts are more or less like clouds that come and go in a big sky. It's difficult to predict what clouds will be floating through our minds this week, let alone in five minutes.

By thinking about the question, *"What will your next thought be?"* you're allowing yourself to leave your mind for a few moments and experience thoughtlessness – which is wonderful. It's like a mental vacation.

After you've tried to answer that question, observe what thoughts actually do pop into your mind. Observe them like you would clouds in a sky. You'll witness that you're not your thoughts, which are often fantasy and not based in the present moment.

The goal of porn is to send you an endless amount of fictitious thoughts; so many that you actually believe they're part of your being. Thoughts are not real.

*10 minutes of silence and focused breathing. Repeat the mantra: "***I don't exist in fantasy. I am present. I am real.***"

Day 4

Exercise:

Observe your body. Observe how it feels, moves, and reacts.

Remember that most people use pornography to bring about an orgasm, or a general feeling of excitement that releases certain neurochemicals in the brain. Many people do this because they're stressed, depressed, or anxious – the world we live in can be taxing on the body, and porn offers the viewer a way to cope. That way involves manipulation of brain chemicals, often produced by the orgasm.

If you're still using pornography today, observe your body movements, sounds, sensations, and breaths during your use of it. Do your eyes look down or roll? Do you move your hands fast or slow? Is there a stopping and starting at certain intervals? Are your fingers clicking a keyboard quickly, slowly? How is your posture? Try to observe everything about your body while viewing porn. Be aware.

If you are not using porn today, then continue with the 10 minutes of silence and focused breathing, but get in touch with your body. A good way to do this is by touching each body part and saying its name, leaving your hand on the part for a few seconds and feeling its texture and warmth. Start with your head: place your hand on your head and say, "*I'm touching my head.*" And then work your way down to your shoulders, arms, stomach, legs, knees, and feet. Focus your attention on one body part at a time.

*10 minutes of silence and focused breathing. Repeat the mantra: "***I am not my body.**"

Day 5

Exercise:

On a piece of paper, write down all the labels and adjectives that you and others use to identify you.

For example, do you see yourself as a son, daughter, mother, father, student, teacher, engineer, accountant, employee, employer, roommate, husband, wife, etc? And what adjectives do you use to label yourself; for example, do you identify yourself as failed, successful, happy, depressed, good, moral, unethical, lustful, greedy, valuable, worthless, etc? Don't only write down the labels and descriptions; but also write down what you believe others see in terms of labels and adjectives. Do you think others see you as a valuable friend, stupid student, incompetent employee, sexy girlfriend, smart person, etc?

Take as long as you need, and fill up a sheet of paper with those labels and descriptions.

After you've done that, tear the paper into multiple pieces and throw it away. Those labels and adjectives mean nothing. They're not "you." You cannot be defined, labeled, described, or controlled. What you wrote on the paper are mere words, and most people poison their conscience with such learned vocabulary. They really believe in these words – they'll even fight, stress, get sick, and die to make these words a reality. Porn, as well as most societal tools, teaches you to identify with particular words, which are only thoughts.

*10 minutes of silence and focused breathing. Repeat the mantra: "**I am not a label, title, or thought.**"

Day 6

Exercise:

Stand still for 5 minutes; with knees slightly bent (i.e. your legs should not be locked). At first try to remain still, but then let your body sway. Let it move any way it wishes. Feel its movement. If you're unable to stand, you can do this same exercise by extending your arm or leg from a sitting position – try to keep it straight, but then let go of trying and allow movement to happen.

We tend to lock ourselves into particular goals, expectations, thought patters, and habits. We even go so far as to be proud of rigidity – people mistake rigidity for perseverance. This is taught to us by our culture. Everything around you may be shouting, even in a quiet whisper, that you must remain submissive and obedient.

Porn, like most dependencies, is no different in its message. It wants you to remain rigid; not to be released from its hold. If you freely moved on from porn use, it would lose you as a customer and dependent. By the way, who wants to remain rigidly dependent on something like porn for their happiness? Or I should say…false happiness.

The message of porn essentially says, "*Stay here with these images and videos. Return to them daily. Use them to your advantage. You need them for sexual fulfillment and comfort.*" Allow your body and mind to move on from porn dependency. Trust that your body and mind will sway to its own rhythm, and away from porn.

*10 minutes of silence and focused breathing. Repeat the mantra: "*I am now free to move. I am free to move on.*"

Day 7

Exercise:

Count to 25 slowly, pausing for a few seconds before the next number; then, count backward from 25 slowly. Try this with your eyes closed.

Our world today is about speed. Everyone seems to be in a rush, yet most of them are unsatisfied; and, they have no clue where they're going. Chasing the next best thing is a fruitless endeavor. It's the rare person who slows down to enjoy the present moment, regardless of the nature of the moment. Because there seems to be so many problems, and most jobs are focused on resolving those problems, people are compelled to accept anxiety and rush toward a reward and conclusion. That surely isn't happiness, because happiness can only be found in the present moment, not in a hypothetical future of reward or success.

The creators of porn know this fact well, so they display the images and videos on technological platforms that allow for this constant demand to rush. How many times have you rushed through porn videos to find the one that matches your desired narrative? This is destructive to your peace of mind and health: concentration suffers, stress levels rise, and awareness to the present moment isn't possible.

It's critical to slow down. You only have one life to live – don't rush through it, and don't be dependent on anything that encourages you to rush.

*10 minutes of silence and focused breathing. Repeat the mantra: "***Slow down. Do not rush. Enjoy the present moment.***"

Day 8

Exercise:

On a piece of paper (any size) write down the goals that you've been striving to achieve – i.e. the goals that you believe will bring you fulfillment. For example: a new job, a house in a nice neighborhood, traveling the world, a business, a family, new friends, a degree or certification, building a network, reaching a net worth of a million dollars, etc.

Now, tear up the paper into multiple pieces, and throw away.

Goals can be very helpful and useful if they're not obsessed over. However, in western culture people develop a reliance on goals. Think about all the times you've said something like, "*I need to get that,*" "*I must reach this,*" "*I'll do anything to accomplish that*", etc. It's often the case that people spend more time worrying about their goals, than freely doing something in the present moment to reach them. Plus, the goal in itself is fleeting, while the journey in the present moment is real and lasting.

The habit of thinking that goals must be met or else failure ensues is subtly applied to dependencies. When you've viewed porn in the past, what was the goal? What was it that you felt you needed to achieve?

*10 minutes of silence and focused breathing. Repeat the mantra: "**My happiness does not depend on meeting a goal. I'm happy now.**"

Day 9

Exercise:

Spend 5 minutes smelling something aromatic: a piece of fruit, a spice, tea, pine, cedar, a flower, a scented candle, etc. Focus on the smell of that one thing for the entire 5 minutes. Don't let anything distract you from the smell.

How often do you take time to enjoy a fragrant smell? One of the lies of modern society is that if you stop and enjoy your five senses too long, you'll miss out on...fill in the blank. While people are rushing toward their goals with stress levels spiking, they're totally missing out on awareness in the present moment. People stare at images of food that others have posted on the internet, but don't take the time to smell or taste food in the present moment.

What's better: watching two actors having sex in an online fantasy, or enjoying the smell of vanilla, orange, or pine in the present reality? The first is fake and illusory; the second is real and sensational. Porn does a great job from stealing time and energy from your other senses, such as smell. One of the best ways get into the present moment and away from an illusion is through focusing on smell and the use of your other senses. Don't let porn diminish your other senses any longer.

*10 minutes of silence and focused breathing. Repeat the mantra: *"I can sense the present."*

Day 10

Exercise:

Focus on a natural object or scene for 10 minutes, without distraction and in silence.

Focusing on a natural object for an extended period of time is an ancient practice. How often have you stopped to observe something objectively for more than 10 minutes? When was the last time you've quietly watched a sunset, sunrise, tree sway in the wind, bird chirping, clouds passing or expanding, or just a rock? That might sound boring, but this practice is very liberating. If you look at anything long enough you start to see it from a different perspective. As easy as this exercise sounds, it's not – try it out, and see how long you can observe without thoughts impeding the practice.

Watching a bird feed may be more interesting than watching an immobile rock; but I encourage you to start with an immobile object, such as a stone or piece of wood. During this process thoughts will emerge – observe the thoughts and let them pass.

Who looks at porn as a mystic would look at a stone? Nobody does; because porn isn't natural. Porn producers don't want you to objectively see the illusion that they're actors who are uncomfortably and deceptively having sex. The purpose of porn is to hypnotize you with a false narrative; stealing your attention from the present.

*10 minutes of silence and focused breathing. Repeat the mantra: "**Be focused. Observe. Be present.**"

Day 11

Exercise:

Imagine being a porn star in the any of the porn films that you've favored.

Have you ever seriously considered what porn actors and actresses think and feel while on the set or in the studio? Take a moment, and put yourself in their shoes.

Imagine that a friend called you, and said, *"Hey, I have a great job for you. You'll make a thousand dollars for twelve hours of work. It's a porn shoot. We need you to fill in for someone."* Now, imagine actually saying yes, showing up to the studio, apartment, hotel room, or wherever it's being shot, and following the orders of the producer: *"Stand there," "You don't look like you're in pain. Look like you're in pain," "Stop. Stop! Change positions. Grab their head. Come on. We don't have all day," "Now scream like you're having the greatest orgasm ever," "Not like that. Do it over," "Ok everyone, we'll have to repeat this again using a different camera and angle."*

Do you think you'll be able to enjoy that work? Despite making a lot of money, would it be fun? And think of the narrative that the film is promoting: a stepfather and stepdaughter situation, a teen and teacher scenario, an unwanted gang bang, a punishment and abuse story, etc. The only person enjoying porn is the dependent viewer…and that's a fleeting enjoyment that evolves in strange ways. It's a twisted perception of reality.

*10 minutes of silence and focused breathing. Repeat the mantra: "**Fantasy is not reality. Reality is here and now.**"

Day 12

Exercise:

If you can stand, stand on one foot and try to stay balanced as long as possible. If you're unable to stand, balance a pen on your wrist or index finger, trying not to let it fall.

Now let your elevated foot, or the balanced pen, drop. Don't force the drop, just let it happen naturally.

All abnormal dependencies want you to balance them with necessary dependencies (eating, drinking, breathing, moving, sensing, etc). Porn doesn't want you to consider it abnormal or damaging to your baseline happiness. It wants you to believe that you can keep it in balance with your basic needs for survival. This is an effective lie of the dependency; and in fact, all dependencies use this lie to keep you hooked.

Understand that porn dependency doesn't help you at all; even in a balanced state. Let's say a person can balance porn with their responsibilities to care for family, work, and staying healthy. The person is fooling themselves, and the porn is slowly but surely taking from present moment awareness. It would be better if this person let the balance fail and watch porn drop to either side – that is, either completely impacting their lives negatively (many call this *hitting rock bottom*) or letting it pass away, like a dark cloud passing in a blue sky.

*10 minutes of silence and focused breathing. Repeat the mantra: "**It is okay to let go. I can let go.**"

Day 13

Exercise:

On a sheet of paper (any size) write down all the internal lies that you regularly hear about yourself – i.e. within your mind.

Now, tear the paper into multiple pieces, and throw away.

It's common to have an internal voice (or voices) within your mind, playing a record of lies over and over. We eventually begin to accept these lies and let them impact our growth and happiness. Most people you see on a daily basis have these recurring internal voices; and most people are oblivious to them – sort of like white noise. This isn't a mental illness, but a way in which the mind works. We all experience these internal quiet voices whispering untruths about our being. These lies are nothing to fear, but need to be observed. Writing them down helps you observe and become aware of their deceptions.

The power of the silence, focused breathing, and mantras, which you have been practicing, is to draw out the lies. Let them manifest, and observe them. Common internal lies include: *"You are a loser," "You have become nothing, and you will never improve," "You are worthless. No one likes you," "You'll always be alone," "You're a burden,"* and so on. These thoughts are not part of you; however, the deception is to make you believe they are. Like many things in our culture, porn implants many of these lies clandestinely.

*10 minutes of silence and focused breathing. Repeat the mantra: **"Thoughts are only thoughts - nothing more."**

Day 14

Exercise:

For 10 minutes, look at your face in a mirror. Analyze its curvature, look closely at the color of your eyes, notice the blemishes and spots, observe its movements, etc. Look at your face as if you were observing someone else's. Do this without judgment, but observe any thoughts that emerge.

Did you experience judgment? Were you upset? Was this an uncomfortable exercise? Were you content with the look of your face? Did any thoughts appear?

Rarely do we stop to look at our faces in a mirror for an extended period of time. You may for a quick moment while cleaning or dressing, but hardly long enough to see its uniqueness. The face may be the most important part of your body, since it's what people recognize most. However, the face that you have is not "you".

Judgment runs rampant today. Even those who say, "*I don't judge. I never judge a person*" are fooling themselves. It takes a lot of practice and mindfulness to be judgment free. It's possible to reach that awareness, but it needs to start with your perception of "you". The day you stop judging yourself, you'll stop judging others.

The hope of porn is that you will diligently judge yourself, consciously and subconsciously, so that you'll seek validation within the confines of its illusory narrative.

*10 minutes of silence and focused breathing. Repeat the mantra: **"I am not my face or body. I do not need validation."**

Day 15

Exercise:

Light a candle and observe its flame for 5 minutes. Watch it move and feel its heat. Appreciate its energy.

Now, blow out the flame.

(If you don't have a candle, light a match and blow it out; and if you don't have a candle or match, stare at a dim light for 5 minutes and then turn it off.)

The temperature of a small candle flame (and match flame) is around 1200 Celsius (which is about 2000 Fahrenheit). That's a lot of energy! And within a fraction of a second, it was extinguished as you blew it out; or in the case of the light, turned off its energy source. There wasn't a gradual process with delays and stops. You blew out the highly energized flame, and that was it - from 1200 Celsius to nonexistent in no time...or should I say in present no time.

We think that our dependencies have so much energy and power. It's not just porn, but all dependencies survive on this deception of power. The truth is that dependencies don't have energy like the candle flame, though your mind may have been tricked into believing they do. The candle flame is real and powerful; whereas dependencies are illusory and fictitious.

As easily and quickly as you distinguished the flame, you can drop a dependency in the present moment.

*15 minutes of silence and focused breathing. Repeat the mantra: "**Dependency isn't real. It is extinguished.**"

Day 16

Exercise:

Taste something by eating it very slowly for at least 5 minutes. Pick something with a lot of flavor: a piece of fruit, a strong tea, a spice, soup with many ingredients, honey, etc. Close your eyes through most of your tasting. Savor the piece of food slowly. Pay close attention to the feel of the taste on your tongue. Chew slowly.

Porn does a great job at stealing presence away from our other senses, as does many dependencies. Since porn is directly related to our reproductive senses, the more those senses are abused the more our other senses are neglected. When was the last time you thoroughly enjoyed the taste of an orange, vanilla, dark chocolate, olive oil, or cheese? I don't mean enjoying the flavor for a few seconds and then continuing on with your meal, but to let the flavor linger before taking another bite.

The taste of a pineapple, pepper, grape, or apple is far more real and satisfying than pornography. It may sound silly to say that, but it's true, because those foods are based in reality. You can actually interact with them in the present, and they don't hypnotize you into an illusory relationship based on neurochemical reliance (the reliance I'm referring to is the orgasm that porn manipulates).

Let the taste of food bring you into the present moment.

*15 minutes of silence and focused breathing. Repeat the mantra: "***I am free to taste.***"

Day 17

Exercise:

Listen to a person intently without interruption. Only speak if the person asks you a question, but don't give a long answer. Make the conversation entirely theirs. Give them the floor, and listen to every word they are saying. Again, do not interrupt. Observe their words and facial expressions without judgment. Be patient and relaxed, even if they speak for more than a few minutes.

Patience is a dying practice in our digital age. It appears that all business involves the perceived need to go faster, faster, and faster. Quicker responses, faster uploads, more data, rapid analysis, accelerated transportation, and all sorts of chop-chop. This false need for speed has seeped deep into our collective psyche. The western world is filled with anxiously demanding people, going nowhere fast.

This widespread lack of patience has caused a problem with regard to listening to one another. It has also caused dependency on porn to manifest extensively. People who are dependent on porn usually don't use one or two images to satisfy their cravings; they click, upload, and download multiple images or videos, and they require this action to happen at lightning speed. Practicing patience by listening intently to someone speak is a great way to slow the mind down and build meaningful relationships. The fabricated relationship of porn cannot compete with real human interaction, which requires patience.

*15 minutes of silence and focused breathing. Repeat the mantra: "**Listen. Be patient. Listen.**"

Day 18

Exercise:

Turn off your cell phone, or put it in airplane mode, for at least 1 hour, and observe the thoughts you experience. If you don't have any major responsibilities this day, or if you have all you need and don't require the phone, then turn off your cell phone for 12 hours. This exercise works best if you can go 24 hours without your cell phone activated; but go no less than 1 hour. If there are people who are immediately dependent on you, send them a text saying that you'll be unavailable, and then turn off your phone.

Like never before in history, we live in a modern world with a plethora of distractions. These distractions fight for our attention, because money is behind the scenes. Every business is wondering how they can break your distraction from one thing so that you can be distracted by their thing – whether that thing is a product or service, such as porn. It's a constant war between everyone. Whoever can hold your attention the longest, wins the battle; but whoever can make you dependent, wins the war.

The porn industry needs for you to be distracted by its business; otherwise you might wake up to reality and enjoy the beauty of life, which includes real sex. Porn has made its way into smartphones; so no longer does the porn dependent viewer need a computer to get off. The dependent can carry porn around and access it at will, strengthening the dependency along the way.

*15 minutes of silence and focused breathing. Repeat the mantra: "*I am not distracted. I am present, here, and now.*"

Day 19

Exercise:

Clean something slowly. Take your time; don't rush the cleaning, and be thorough. You can clean your room, car, kitchen, bathroom, bag, desk drawer, shoes...anything. Go slow, and give full attention to what you're doing. Throw away as much stuff as possible.

Though most of us hate cleaning and only do it when the mess has become monstrous, cleaning is known to be therapeutic for a reason. We attach to our clutter fairly quickly, but we don't enjoy it. Regular cleaning is a wonderful practice because we're letting go of disorder in the present moment, in a very practical way.

Similar to a messy kitchen that can look depressing; the mind can experience depression because of pornographic clutter. Remember that porn is an illusion, so the person who utilizes porn regularly is filling the mind and body with misconceptions and fantasies that block authentic perception in the present moment. The only way to clear this type of unseemly mental clutter is through observation, understanding, and awareness.

The exercises in this book are purposed to help clear your mind from the mess that porn leaves, so you can perceive clearly. If you haven't experienced it already, waking up to a life without porn dependency is refreshing and exciting.

*15 minutes of silence and focused breathing. Repeat the mantra: *"I am clean. My mind is clear."*

Day 20

Exercise:

Hold a smile for 5 minutes. You don't need to do this exercise in front of a mirror; but feel free to do so if you wish. You can even do this exercise during the 15 minutes of silence and focused breathing. While holding your smile, take a moment and feel your face; actually touch the smile and the curvature of your lips and cheek bones.

Have you ever behaved a certain way and then saw your mood change immediately? Physical exercise, such as running and weightlifting, does this for many people. Certain forms of yoga have also been used by people to change their moods. The point is: changing your behavior not only impacts other people, but can also impact your perception.

You'll notice that while you're smiling during this exercise, you may experience certain emotions. You might feel silly, embarrassed, stupid, funny, weird, or whatever. Continue smiling regardless. In fact, if you are still using porn at this point in the program, smile while you're viewing it – hold the smile until you are through with your porn use. As always, observe your thoughts while you're smiling; observe the thoughts as if they're clouds passing by in a bright blue sky.

Smiling causes an authentic reaction in our bodies and minds that is essentially good. The present moment enjoys a nice smile. So hold that smile until you no longer can.

*15 minutes of silence and focused breathing. Repeat the mantra: *"**Happiness is now. I am happy.**"*

Day 21

Exercise:

Choose a physical symbol that will remind you to observe and be aware in the present moment. Try to choose something from nature, or that is made of natural material.

The object you choose can be anything, but it's best if it's something that you can enjoy looking at and touching. For example, many walkers and hikers will find a unique rock small enough to carry in their hands. A stone, necklace, bracelet, seashell, cedar block, coin…anything will do, as long as you enjoy it and you can dedicate it as a tool for remembrance.

Another cunning trick of porn is to confuse the mind into forgetting you're part of the natural world. Porn requires you to use the imagination, which can be easily manipulated for the business of porn. Thus, you're taken out of physical reality. By having a symbol of remembrance, you can reconnect with the present moment. This symbol isn't meant to be an idol, god, or icon. Don't think too deeply into this. The symbol is simply a tool to help you remember where you are in the *here and now*. As long as you're aware of the present, you'll have no desire to return to the hallucination of porn.

*15 minutes of silence and focused breathing. Repeat the mantra: "***All is well. Here and now, all is well.***"

Day 22

Exercise:

On a sheet of paper (one that you can easily save and return to later) make a list of hobbies that you've had in the past but have neglected, and also make a list of hobbies that you would like to start in the future.

From these lists choose one hobby from the past and one new hobby that you'd like to start. Focus only on these two – the old hobby and the new one. Make this a priority.

How often have you said, or have heard other people say, "*I wish I had the time.*" You do have the time. You just choose to think of time in the way that you've been taught to perceive it. If your life depended on it, you would certainly make the time if needed.

In fact, time is a manmade construct…don't ever forget that. There is only ever the present moment. Past and future are not here and now. We spend far too much time thinking about time. How many of your recurrent inner thoughts involve questions such as, "*When will that ever happen?*" "*When will I ever change?*" "*Why did that have to happen?*" "*If the past was different, life would be better.*" These are lies that only eat into the present moment, and infect our modern world.

Porn occupies the present moment; and that moment could be used to pursue hobbies that magnify your happiness.

*15 minutes of silence and focused breathing. Repeat the mantra: "**The time is now. It is the present moment.**"

Day 23

Exercise:

Deliberately feel the sensation of water on your skin for at least 5 minutes. You can do this exercise in the shower, while washing your hands, taking a bath, going for a swim, walking in the rain, or simply placing your hand in a sink filled with water. Close your eyes if you like.

How often do you deliberately experience the essence of water? We take it for granted every day. It's a remarkable chemical substance in the universe that is necessary for all life. Without it, we wouldn't exist. This one transparent and fluid substance has immense capacity. A large percentage of your physical body is made of this natural substance. Experience it.

Every day we jump in the shower, wash our hands, and drink it – but rarely do we take time to slowly and deliberately appreciate our natural response to water. Porn can never give you the energy, sensation, reality, and present moment that water can give. Water is an example of a positive dependency that doesn't bind you emotionally or spiritually. Water doesn't need you; porn, however, does.

There are many lessons that water can teach: fluidity, flow, evaporation, change, motion, stillness, and life. You can't get any of those lessons through an illusion such as porn, or any unnatural dependency for that matter.

*15 minutes of silence and focused breathing. Repeat the mantra: *"I am fluid. I change. I flow."*

Day 24

Exercise:

Say the words "Guilt", "Shame", and "Regret" 10 times to yourself out loud. Don't rush. Pause between each repetition. For the pause, you can take a deep breath. Your eyes can remain open or closed. Again, don't rush - say the words slowly and observe any thoughts, feelings, or images that emerge internally.

Now, say these words again 10 times, but with a smile.

What futile credence we give words such as Guilt, Shame and Regret. We use these words on ourselves as well as others; they become regular vocabulary for our internal recurring voices. And in the end, they're mere words that hold no power. What would these words be without a facial expression, tone, inflection, or emphasis?

When you said these three specific words, what thoughts came to mind, what did you feel, and was there a reaction in your body? If there was a reaction, such as shortness of breath or a frown, people tend to interpret it as sadness; but this reaction is a learned behavior. We've been taught to feel and think a certain way with regard to guilt, shame, and regret. The truth is: these words mean nothing.

Porn, like most dependencies, flourishes on these three words and the learned reactions they produce. But see them for that they are…mere words with no power.

*15 minutes of silence and focused breathing. Repeat the mantra: "**I am not Guilt. I am not Shame. I am not Regret.**"

Day 25

Exercise:

On a piece of paper (any size) write down the name of your current emotion. For example, at this moment you might be feeling agitated, calm, bored, angry, anxious, excited, etc. Whatever emotion you are experiencing, give it a name and put it on paper.

Now, write down "I'm experiencing this emotion in the present moment and it will pass. It's only an emotion."

You can throw the paper away, or hold onto it if you wish.

Similar to how we give certain words credence, we tend to give our emotions a lot of trust. We also tend to blame the outside world for emotions we are feeling: *"They made me angry," "I'm depressed because they didn't want me," "If they gave me the job, I would be happy."*

The emotions you feel are in you, not in the outer world. No one can cause you to feel or emote in a particular way; if they're able to, it's only because you let them. A great way to let a harmful emotion pass is to observe it; and a good start is by giving it a name and seeing it as powerless.

It's commonplace to blame others for our pain. Instead of seeing the emotion for what it is and letting it pass, we've been taught to rely on dependencies, like porn, to manage the emotional reaction. Wake up! Emotions are not you.

*15 minutes of silence and focused breathing. Repeat the mantra: *"I am not an emotion. All emotions that I experience will pass."*

Day 26

Exercise:

Today, look for the color blue in your surrounding environment. If possible, spend the entire day looking for the color blue in the places you go. Whether you're doing this exercise in a bedroom, office, classroom, outside, or while traveling, look for the color blue in all things that surround you. If you think you'll forget to do this throughout the entire day, spend at least 20 focused minutes practicing this exercise at some point.

Focused attention is something that must be practiced - it doesn't come easy in our rapid paced society. Instead of encouraging us to focus and observe, the modern world encourages us to rush and get things done.

Searching for a color or shape helps to slow down our accelerated and cyclical thought patterns, and reminds us that there's more to the world than the chaotic thoughts we collectively and daily experience. By searching for the color blue, your mind can escape the fictitious grip of anxiety, lust, desire, depression, worry, fear, or any other potent emotion. When you were using porn, were you aware of the colors in the film or image? Most likely not.

Porn functions to distract your conscience from present reality. Look for the color blue today, and wake up to life in the present moment.

*15 minutes of silence and focused breathing. Repeat the mantra: "*I am focused, here and now.*"

Day 27

Exercise:

Make yourself laugh for 5 minutes. Don't stop laughing. You might feel strange, weird, embarrassed, or stupid...it doesn't matter, just laugh. Try to laugh alone and without the aid of a comedy or joke. If you don't know how to start, just start making the noises that typically accompany your laughter.

What feelings did you experience during this exercise? Many people report feeling embarrassed or goofy, which is great; however, most people also report a feeling of relief and buoyancy when they've completed this exercise.

Similar to holding a smile, laughing for 5 minutes is a fantastic way to come into present awareness. If you think about it, humor is necessary for life. How sad is the person who is unable to laugh at the experiences of life? After all, life is funny.

If you ever experience the desire to use porn again, simply laugh at it. Consider how porn is idiotic and frivolous; it really is a funny dependency. No other living thing on the planet becomes dependent on watching naked bodies bang for bucks. It's quite stupid, and thus funny. If you perceive porn for what it truly is - a fictitious, impractical, and frivolous imagery – then it can be easily dropped.

*15 minutes of silence and focused breathing. Repeat the mantra: **"Life is wonderful, funny, and real."**

Day 28

Exercise:

Look at a picture or painting for 10 minutes, alone, in silence, and without any distraction. It would be best if the picture isn't of family or friends, but it could have been created by someone you know. Try to choose a work of art for this exercise, but any picture or painting will suffice.

Porn isn't art; though some people will argue it is – those people are typically arguing in order to hold onto the dependency. Porn producers, directors, and actors aren't making pornography for the purpose of art; instead, they're making it to capitalize off peoples' dependencies. Despite porn being image based, have you ever seen porn advertised as art?

When images of pornography occupy the mind, there's a loss of connection to images that can be helpful to the awakened mind. The purpose of this exercise is to return the mind to an appreciation of truly inventive and innovative art. A printed picture hanging in a cheap motel room has more artistry than the most popular trending porn film.

Observing a picture, photo, or print for an extended period of time can aid the mind in slowing down. You may have had a photo of a landscape hanging in your home for many years, but have you ever taken the time to carefully analyze it? Take some time and do that. Appreciate the image, and observe your thoughts in the process.

*15 minutes of silence and focused breathing. Repeat the mantra: **"Stillness. Silence. Peace. Presence."**

Day 29

Exercise:

Go for a mindfulness walk for at least 10 minutes. Focus on each step. Feel the steps: the feel of your feet hitting the ground, your heel rolling forward, your toes, the bend of your knees, your hips working to balance your posture, the swinging of your arms, etc. Don't rush; go slow. Focus on your breathing as well. Get in tune with your body as you step. Pay attention to your physical senses throughout the walk. Focus – don't listen to music or be distracted.

Human beings have always used walking as a natural therapeutic exercise. There is something about walking, and focusing on the walk, that calms the mind and soul. The longer one walks, the more relaxed the person feels.

Any moment is a good time to walk and experience your inner and outer environment. During long walks, thoughts will emerge that will allow you to graciously observe them. Let the thoughts pass; you may even have emotions that emerge, observe those and let them pass as well. Focusing on your steps will help you clear the mind of clutter. Walking in the early morning and at dusk is especially beneficial.

A 20 minute walk brings more comfort, stillness, peace, focus, and awareness than thousands of hours of using porn. Walk every day, as much as you can.

*15 minutes of silence and focused breathing. Repeat the mantra: "*I am relaxed. I am at peace.*"

Day 30

Exercise:

One last time, take a piece of paper (one that you can keep) and write down all that you are grateful for – these things don't have to be in any particular order of importance.

Next to each thing you list, write "Thank you."

Strong dependencies don't encourage gratitude. The person who isn't thankful for all that life gives is typically quite miserable, and dependencies flourish on that misery. The truly grateful person can let go at any time. A thankful person is a happy person.

Have you ever heard anyone say, *"I'm so grateful for porn! I wrote a letter to the producer of my favorite film, thanking him for his hard work. I also contacted the actors and marketers and thanked them for benefiting my life."* Nobody is thankful for porn; which is a clear sign that it's a destructive dependency.

Not only is it unhealthy, but porn doesn't encourage a grateful mind and soul. With only one life to live in the present moment, it's important to always emphasize a grateful heart. Spend time with people who are grateful, and do things that encourage a thankful heart. Anything that causes misery and depression, such as porn use, isn't worth giving attention to.

*15 minutes of silence and focused breathing. Repeat the mantra: *"I am grateful. I am thankful."*

Conclusion

If you've made it through the 30 days, that's wonderful! Whether you sense it or not, you have developed some amazing skills that you can carry into other areas of your life. All that we experience is in the present moment, and to be reliant on an unhealthy dependency isn't a good use of the present. Hopefully you've dropped your dependency and moved on to more valuable experiences.

If there were any particular exercises, lessons, and mantras that helped you the most, pay close attention to those. I encourage you to continually practice the ones that have been most beneficial to you. I also want to encourage you to modify the exercises as well as create your own, tailored to your present experience. No two people are the same. As you grow into awareness and free from dependency, your practices will evolve and you'll gain liberation.

Enjoy freedom from porn dependency, and don't bother looking back. Stay grounded in the present moment.

Made in the USA
Coppell, TX
08 January 2025